# Go To The

# GYM

## CHRIS JANKE-BUENO

# CONTACT CHRIS

Contact us at My Core Balance by phone or through our website.

408-883-4442

www.MyCoreBalance.com

# CONTENTS


Momentum is your #1 "Muscle"    1

Why Do We Procrastinate?    10

Change Your Mindset    15

Take Action    24

Course Correction    38

# ACKNOWLEDGMENTS

I'd like to thank all my cheerleaders, those friends, family, and clients who have supported me and my book writing.

# CHAPTER 1
# MOMENTUM IS YOUR #1 NUMBER GOAL

Usually when we think about exercise, we think about muscles. We think about cardio. We think about core training. But what if exercise was all about developing your habits?

You've likely done research online, and googled something like "what's the best workout program" or "how to exercise properly" or something like that. The goal of this book is to get you thinking more in terms of consistency first, and then focus on what to do next.

Momentum is the number one "muscle" that you want to build. Think about it. How many times have you "tried" a fitness program, yet stopped doing it after several weeks, or worse yet maybe several days?

No shame, no guilt. We've all done it. In my 15 years as a personal trainer, I have seen that if people just spend a little bit more effort on establishing habits and thinking about maintaining momentum, then they won't get derailed and lose their results.

If we were to break this down percentagewise, it might be something like 80% of your focus needs to be on establishing good habits. 20% (or less!) needs to be on figuring out which program you actually want to do. If you are going to hire a personal trainer, that percentage will be even less than 20%, even zero!

The number one "muscle" that you want to begin cultivating is the power of daily practice. It doesn't matter what you do, it just matters that you do something.

Several years ago, I learned this firsthand. I made the goal to show up to the gym every day for 30 days. I didn't make the goal to exercise every day, I just made the goal to show up. It was achievable, it was winnable.

I very easily completed this goal, despite a few days out of those 30 I simply showed up to the gym, went in the sauna, took a shower and left. But that was a victory. I made a very achievable goal, and after the 30 days I had a huge amount of momentum.

You too can create this momentum. Momentum starts with one baby step. That baby step turns into 30 baby steps which will constitute your kickstarting month.

One healthy month can create enough momentum to last for years.

So let's work on creating your first month, building some momentum so that you can win with your health and fitness goals.

## Being Realistic About The Time It Takes To Achieve A Fitness Goal

A long weekend is not a long enough time to devote to achieving a fitness goal. In a long weekend you may be able to come up with a plan, but the implementation of that plan takes months or even years.

If you do a Google search, you will find that people will disagree slightly, but they are all in the general ballpark. One to two pounds per week is a healthy amount of body fat to lose if you are doing everything right. Meaning you're exercising hard enough and you are eating well.

So on the conservative end we are looking at four pounds per month. But I've definitely seen people lose 10 or so pounds in a month. A lot of this depends on how much you have to lose.

Let's take a step back here. The actual process of losing weight is really not hard. What it takes is making the decision to follow a certain path. Once you start following a path, then it's just a matter of putting one foot in front of the other.

I'm simply talking here about a mindset shift. Putting most of your energy into the upfront momentum building, and cultivating these habits. Since you know you're going to be in this for the long term, you can take your time and work on building these habits, which will in turn create results.

Another common goal is for people to want to gain muscle mass. Gaining muscle is even slower than losing fat, if you're looking simply at pounds. It takes about a month to gain one pound of muscle. If you want to gain 10 pounds of muscle, you are looking at probably one year of hard training and good nutrition.

Set your mind and your energy into creating the habits that will create the body for you. There's probably only a handful of habits that healthy people do. Work on cultivating more of those habits.

These habits are not overnight things. You can't just do one workout and expect success. It takes months to years to achieve your results.

The next step I recommend that you think about is what I call the *doubling effect*. However much time you think it will take to reach your goals, I want you to double that number. I want you to allow yourself that much time to achieve your goals.

This doubling effect is not necessarily inspiring. It's not going to sell the latest and greatest "secret" new exercise equipment on QVC. But it works because it's the truth. And it takes pressure off of your back and allows you to be real about the timetable to fitness.

Start telling yourself the truth about how long this is actually going to take you, because that is the first step toward actual success with your health and fitness program.

## We Are All Creatures Of Habit

Let's start with a simple example that is pretty obvious. When was the last time you thought about tying your shoe? I mean given real conscious thought to the act of tying your shoe. If I were to guess, it's probably been a long time.

Yet, your shoes get tied every day. Who ties your shoes? Well, obviously you do. But you don't think about tying your shoes. So how does it get done.

As simple as that above example is, I challenge you to think of your fitness goals in the same way. If you are not as healthy and fit as you want to be, it's only because you haven't made going to the gym as habitual as tying your shoes. End of story. That's it.

The examples are many. Tying your shoes, driving a car, getting dressed in the morning, taking a shower... You have dozens of routines that you do on a daily, weekly, and monthly basis. Let's put "going to the gym" or "running around the neighborhood" at the top of the list.

For years, and even decades, I looked for the "secret sauce" of fitness. I wanted to know if there was a special **program** that works better than the others.

There's not.

I wanted to know if there's a certain **protocol** that's better than the others.

There's not.

With fitness, there are no secrets. Sure, There are certain principles that should be followed. But they are not that complicated. There is no secret. There's just consistency.

Let me ask you something. Fast forward to today's date one year from now. If you can look back on the previous year and say that you had created a new habit of going to the gym every day, how much better do you think your life would be? Regardless of how much weight you actually lost.

Regardless of how much muscle you actually gained. If you take the next year and really develop the habit of exercising every day, how much better would your life be?

As simple as it sounds, the first step really is to acknowledge that you're number one fitness goal should be to develop the habit of fitness. It's not about the end result. The end result comes from months or years of fine-tuning your approach. But the first prerequisite is just to show up every single day.

Hopefully you agree that this is the number one goal, let's talk about some ways that we can begin to implement that goal.

# CHAPTER 2
# WHY DO WE PROCRASTINATE?

Procrastination is a big ugly word. Even the most efficient and productive people have a tendency to procrastinate at least occasionally. So it helps to address the root causes of procrastination here before we move on.

I believe there are two main causes of procrastination, and they both originate from fear.

***A quick side note about fear, many people say that fear is actually the opposite of love. Not hate, but actually fear.***

The two fears that I'm talking about our first the fear of failure, and second the fear of success.

The fear failure makes a lot of sense. Nobody likes to fail. Nobody likes to fall flat on their face. The second one is a little bit more questionable. Who would have a fear of success? Let me explain both.

You don't want to be a failure. This is a legitimate fear. Nobody wants to fail at something that they set up to do. It's a fear of losing face, losing credibility in a sense. There may be a psychological underpinning of honesty. Think about it, if you say you're going to do something, but it doesn't quite get done exactly how you wanted it to, in a sense, people may fear that they are lying to themselves or others.

This is somewhat understandable. Nobody wants to be a liar. But we need to clarify what this means. Attempting something that you've never attempted Before will inherently bring some risks. It's also 100%

guaranteed that if you've never done something before, you don't know how to do it and therefore you don't know what the future will look like.

Henry David Thoreau said it best: "If one advances confidently in the **direction** of his dreams, and endeavors to live the life which he has imagined, he will meet with a success unexpected in common hours." Don't wait for all the lights to turn green before you start. Just get started today in the **general direction**. You will have plenty of time to modify your approach as needed.

The fear of success is a little bit different. Your success means that you need to stand on your own. People are social creatures. We don't want to be outcasts. When we achieve a big goal, we may leave people behind. What I've found is that this is not true. You can't leave people behind.

Success brings its own issues. I should say the "perception" of success brings its own issues. Zig Ziglar said that you don't pay the price for success, you pay the price for failure. You enjoy the benefits of success.

The fact that so many of us think that somehow our lives will be worse off once we succeed is silly. You can always go back to where you started, you know how to do that.

One great way to mitigate the fear of success is to imagine it every day. The subconscious mind doesn't know the difference between actual Experience and imagined experience. If you imagine achieving your goal often enough and with enough emotion, your success will feel so familiar that your body will naturally start shifting in that direction. It is a slow and gradual process, but it doesn't have to be difficult.

Each of us has a comfort zone similar to a thermostat. If it gets too hot or too cold in the room, the thermostat kicks in and tells the heater or cold air to turn on. Similarly, we have a specific success thermostat. If we get too successful or if we succeed or fail too much according to our own self image, the thermostat kicks on and either brings us down a peg or forces us up.

Sometimes it's hard to believe that we would ever intentionally drop ourselves down. This is a very primitive part of our psychological being. We fear the unknown. The more you meditate, and visualize, the more **known** your future is.

Rehearse your success daily. We will talk about this in a later chapter.

# CHAPTER 3
# CHANGE YOUR MINDSET

## *The Carrot And The Stick*

Human behavior is complicated. Who knows why people do certain things. Sometimes I'm sure you've seen somebody do something and you have to wonder "why the heck did they do that?"

However, despite the fact that human behavior is complicated and nuanced, we can usually break it down into two main drivers: the **carrot** and the **stick**.

The carrot and the stick come from the metaphor of riding on a horse. If you dangle a carrot in front of the horse it will walk forward toward that carrot. On the other hand, if you hit the horse on the butt with a stick it will also walk forward. Both are the same result, but through different means.

People need both carrots and sticks to motivate them. In fact, we are best motivated to take action when there's a healthy combination of both.

The carrot refers to goals, those behaviors that we want… those outcomes that we want to produce or those daily or weekly habits that we want to cultivate. These are the good things that we want more of in our lives.

The "sticks" in our lives are the divorces, the bankruptcies, the car accidents, etc. It could be having to donate $100 to a politician who you don't like.

The stick can be a memory of something that happened to you in the past. Maybe it was a negative outcome that happened after you failed to do something. Of course you don't want to beat yourself over the head with the stick, but it does help sometimes to remember these things because it can help you to take action.

It's vital that you have a combination of carrots (goals, positive habits) and sticks (imagining the worst).

Let's dive a little deeper into the concepts of the carrot and the stick.

## The Carrot - Moving Toward What You Want

It's very important that we all have something compelling and a reason to go for it. This offers us hope and a compelling reason to live.

Do you have goals that are important to you? This is perhaps the number one most important thing when you are setting goals. It's absolutely imperative that your goals are meaningful to you.

If not, you run the risk of basically creating goals that you think other people want you to achieve, which is definitely a very bad place to be. If you have no spark, no drive to achieve your goals, then you will have no energy to do the things you need to do.

What is so important to you that you would risk your life for those achievements? I would argue that this is a prerequisite to achieving anything great. If we're talking about smaller goals, then maybe you won't necessarily die for that goal. But I find that the more you have to lose, the more action you will take.

Think about it, somebody who is facing bank foreclosure on their home will fight like hell to prevent that from happening. Taking a midnight job if they have to, doing whatever it takes.

If a family member is using drugs and destroying their life, doing whatever it takes to get them out of that black hole is necessary.

If you are pursuing a fitness goal that doesn't seem particularly monumental, sometimes it helps to make it bigger than it actually is.

What do I mean by this?

If the "carrot" of a healthy body is not very big and appealing to you, sometimes you can make the carrot bigger. What is important to you? What do you enjoy doing? Maybe you need to associate your fitness goal with some other reward. If having your fitness goal is not intrinsically valuable, maybe you need to give yourself a present after you achieve your goal.

Perhaps you take your family to Disneyland after you lose 50 pounds. Maybe you give $1,000 of your own money to a friend and tell your friend that they can't give it back to you until you lose your weight.

When I was first cultivating the habit of exercising every day I did a few things to "trick" my brain. One very simple one was after I left the gym I would look at the hill about a half a mile away. I live in San Jose, and there are no big mountains nearby unless you drive four hours to Lake Tahoe. But there are small hills surrounding the valley. I left the gym, stood proud, and looked at that hill, which I called Victory Mountain.

I acknowledged Victory Mountain, and that I had just scaled the mountain to the top. I stood like a conqueror. This may seem small, but I really looked forward to Victory Mountain at the end of every workout. I would go into the gym in the dark at 5 AM, and I would emerge an hour and a half later a victor.

Several years ago I heard of a trainer who charged his clients $20,000 upfront to train with him. After every workout he would hand them a $20 bill. Now this is weird. It was their money that they were just getting back, but the psychology behind getting paid to exercise is amazing. This is a great strategy, because if you showed up to every workout all year, you ended up getting a large percentage of your money back... and fitness results too.

You can get leverage on yourself in so many different ways where you **have to** act. If it's a "have to" you will do it. So figure out some creative ways that will force you to act.

## The Stick - Moving Away From What You Don't Want

Now, let's move to the stick. The stick can be even more motivating than the carrot. I think a lot of this depends on how you were raised. If you were punished a lot for misbehavior, the stick might be more real to you than simply having a carrot. It definitely was for me.

I've had dreams of being a writer and producing books for years. But it wasn't until last year that my friend Katie Peuvrelle and I decided to create Product Club.

Katie and I put a challenge to each other. Our goal was to create a product every single month. That was our carrot. Our stick was that if we failed to produce a product by midnight on the last day of the month, we had to donate $100 to a politician who we don't like.

Guess what? Both of us have achieved that goal five months straight and I know that we will not stop soon. Having the combination of the carrot and the stick as allowed both of us to achieve our goals because we are running toward something and simultaneously running away from something else.

Another very practical strategy is using negative imagination in a positive way. It's great to imagine your goals and your reasons for wanting to achieve them. But have you ever imagined what your life is going to be like if you don't achieve your goals?

Fast forward five years and imagine five years from now without having achieved your goal. How would your life be a failure? How would it feel to know that for the last five years you've done nothing in the way of achieving your goals?

Sound harsh? Maybe, but it works. You don't want to go negative and stay there. You want to go negative just long enough to achieve a positive outcome.

The key is that once you know what you don't want, you have to replace that with a compelling vision of what you actually want. The stick by itself doesn't work. The stick creates power, But the carrot creates results.

Think of it like a rocket ship. The explosion is the stick, it gives you the energy and it starts the process. But the aiming system is the carrot. It directs that pure energy to a worthwhile target. Ultimately, you need both!

# CHAPTER 4
# TAKE ACTION

## *Using a habits-based approach*

There are so many things in this world that we cannot control. You can control effort and attitude, but you may not necessarily be able to control results. You can control gym attendance, but you can't control exactly how much weight you lose. I call these two types of goals inputs and outputs.

You can control inputs 100% of the time. However, you cannot control outputs, the best you can hope for is to influence them. For example, you can influence the direction of your goals. You can get healthier. But you can't influence exactly how many pounds you will lose.

Focusing on inputs and your day-to-day habits is important and should take up 80% of your time and attention. Outputs still need a little bit of focus, but the outputs are more like directions.

Hundreds of years ago, when sailing ships were navigating the globe, the captains used the stars to navigate direction. Obviously, they knew that they would never reach the stars. But the stars offered a direction to travel.

Likewise, the outputs are something to reach for, but not necessarily something to touch and hold.

Here's an example from my own fitness journey. My output goals are very specific, yet I also know that I may never touch them fully. My output goals are that I want to weigh 200 pounds, have under 10% body fat, and have 16 inch arms.

However, on a day-to-day basis, I don't focus on this at all. The only time I focus on this is when I'm planning my workouts.

So once I know what I want to achieve, what "star" and going toward, I start to build the program. This is the area where it would be helpful for you to get a personal trainer, because a good trainer will have a very firm grasp about what programs will lead you in what direction.

My program depends on where I am now and where I want to go. Over the last 12 months I've gained about 15 pounds of mass. About 10 of those pounds have been muscle, and I've also gained five pounds of extra fat. Now I'm shifting directions and tweaking my program. My goal now is to maintain the muscle and start slowly losing the fat.

So my daily and weekly routines will be different. My focus now and for the next several months is simply on the inputs of my day-to-day routines.

Using the habit-based approach lets you more accurately determine whether your plan is working.

Here's an example. If you are failing to achieve your goals, yet you have not been consistent with your habit of going to the gym, then there's no way to know if your failure is due to your lack of consistency or if you created a program that doesn't quite match up with your goals.

What if, on the other hand, you have been consistent? Let's say you've been to the gym every day for the last six months. At this point there are only two options. Either you're going in the direction of your goals or you're not.

If you are headed in the right direction, then you know that your plan is good. You may also make subtle tweaks to your program in order to clean up some of the details.

On the other hand, if you have been consistent but you feel like you're going in the complete wrong direction, then your program may need a giant overhaul.

But regardless of whether you are achieving your goals or not, consistency is the prerequisite for determining whether your program is the right one for you at this time. Once you get started you will be able to fine-tune your direction.

## *Plus One Habit Creation*

There are only a handful of habits that you really need to cultivate to become a really fit and healthy person. But even then, sometimes that can seem like a lot.

In order to mitigate this difficulty, I use something called **Plus One Habit Creation**. It's a very simple concept and it works.

Start with the most important habit. It might take you a few days or possibly even a few weeks or months. Once you have mastered the first habit, move onto the next most important habit. Check your progress in any app you want, or you can use a paper calendar, check marks on the wall, whatever. It doesn't matter.

The important thing is that you only focus on one habit at a time. You focus on the most important habit because you have the biggest "bang for your buck" by pursuing that one habit.

Human beings are achievement animals. Checklists work because they offer you a sense of victory every time you complete one part of it.

In my nutrition book **Help! My Diet Sucks!** the entire book is a seven point checklist designed to get your nutrition up to par. Once you've completed your seven steps, then you can get specific with details. The important thing is that you create some momentum behind your nutrition habits.

## *Make A 30-Day Checklist, And Go To The Gym Every Day*

This book is specifically geared toward getting you into the gym every day, cultivating a gym habit that stays with you for the rest of your life. The start of that habit is 30 simple days.

With **Plus One Habit Creation**, your number one task is to go to the gym every day for 30 days. Get started on your journey. Decide where you are going to go every day for the next 30 days. Don't worry about day 31 and beyond. Literally only focus on 30 days.

I would say that you should actually start today, do not even wait until tomorrow. Do you know the old joke "my diet starts on Monday?" That is a horrible way to live. You're always projecting in the future.

Get started today. You're still awake, so you are still here today and you have the chance to be done with day number one. Even if it's 10 PM when you are reading this, you can "get down and give me 20." Call that your first workout of the 30 days.

Allow yourself to build momentum. Allow the law of compounding to benefit you. Going from 0 to 1 takes a lot of work and the result is small. But if you fast forward one year from now, going from 364 to 365 days is the same small step but it was just the final step to one year. Momentum builds and you start to get fitter and healthier.

You can do it!

## *Setting Up Your Support System*

It's vitally important that you surround yourself with people and technology that support you. When you are beginning a new habit you want to cut out everything and everybody that is a drag on you and your goals.

Fitness is an individual endeavor. However, you can get a team around you to help you. Ultimately, you do the work yourself, but you can have people help you with support and encouragement.

I do need to reiterate that ultimately the burden falls on your shoulders because it's true. The recommendations in the next couple of paragraphs serve only to assist you in doing your work. But remember, it is **your** work. Even if you go to the gym with somebody, or even if you hire a personal trainer, you must do the work yourself.

The first step on the accountability ladder is very simple. You can join a gym to give you a place to go. However, the downside of a simple gym membership is that you will not receive a lot of support. If you miss a day, nobody calls. If you miss a week, nobody cares. In fact, the gym industry relies on people like you, people who miss months or even years of workouts but continue to pay their monthly dues. **Don't become one of these people!**

The next step in the accountability ladder would be to get a buddy, an accountability partner who will do the workouts with you. This is very beneficial because most people will break a promise to themselves before they will break a promise to somebody else. So it's less likely that you will break an appointment with this person.

However, sometimes this can turn into "the blind leading the blind." If you don't have the level of fitness that you want, and your friend doesn't either, then nobody really is the "expert" here. If you are both super motivated, this can work. But make sure that neither one of you lets the other off the hook. Never miss a workout.

The next level of accountability is attending a group class. In a group class you have people who get used to seeing you, yet you may not get anybody calling you if you miss a workout. But you will definitely get more customized attention than you would if you just joined a gym.

A way to create a hybrid between an accountability partner and a class is to join a class with a friend. That way you get the benefit of somebody calling you if you don't show up, and also the instruction of somebody who knows what they're doing.

The highest form of accountability is to hire a one-on-one trainer. This person not only will call if you don't show up, but they've also spent some time creating a customized program for you to follow, Which may also include homework for you to do on the days that you're not meeting with your trainer.

The way that I train my clients is sort of a hybrid between personal training and group classes. It's not a drop in class, there is a set schedule, so you have to show up. You have that accountability that you would with a personal trainer. But it's in a small group environment, so you get the benefit of fun, while being accountable to your trainer and classmates. The group environment also brings the price down when compared to traditional one-on-one personal training. And I use an app to issue your homework. 100% accountability.

Now let's talk technology. Pretty much everybody has a smartphone. And if you don't, you may need to use a paper calendar for this. Either way, you'll be fine.

There are tons of apps out there that can help you with this. As a personal preference, I find that the simpler the app the better. If it can send me notifications at certain times, I'm good. I don't necessarily need the most high tech Gantt chart out there, just a calendar system with reminders tends to work for me. But everybody is different. So in this regard, you need to use what works for you.

I've seen people get success from putting a calendar on the wall and marking an X through each date that they go to the gym. This is a powerful visual representation of your progress. You know exactly where you stand with your workouts.

There's something to be said about a large piece of paper hung prominently in your house. Because it's big, you're sending a message that it's important in your life.

Since it's in one set spot in your house, you are guaranteed to see it every day. Whereas information on your phone is small and you may not remember to look at it every day.

## Practical Ways To Stay Motivated

So far I've talked a lot about tracking and showing up. But we haven't talked yet about motivation. What if you start losing the desire to track your progress?

I found that it helps to constantly remind yourself of what you're trying to achieve and why you're trying to achieve it. Remind yourself of your big picture vision.

I have seen people put Vision Boards on their walls, where they glue pictures of what they want to achieve. This works very well. For me, what I have found works even better is to do something called a Mind Movie.

A Mind Movie works because it's multimedia. There's sound, music, video, and words.

If you are skilled at using some of the video editing software that is out there, I recommend making a Mind Movie. Basically, you mix music with your voice saying what you want to achieve and why you want to achieve it. You also add in pictures, videos, and text of your goals. All this comes together to be sort of like a music video of your big picture goals. Pick a song that is the most inspiring for you and keeps you motivated.

Visit
www.MyCoreBalance.com/go-to-the-gym
to see an example of a Mind Movie.

# CHAPTER 5
# COURSE CORRECTION

Course correction is the concept that will save you from going off track and also save you from thinking that going off track is a bad thing. Periodically checking in on a daily, weekly, monthly, quarterly, and yearly basis will ensure that you are headed toward your goals consistently.

## Daily Check-In

The daily check-in is a vital and easy way to make sure you are keeping fuel in your tank. If you only think about your goals on New Year's Day, you've lost the battle. You have too much momentum to overcome and not enough time to do it.

On the other hand, it's important to realize that it doesn't take much, but it does take a daily effort. Unless you discipline yourself on a day-to-day basis to remind yourself of what you want to achieve and why you want to achieve it, you will never get there.

It will take you no more than about 10 minutes per day. Here are some things that I recommend you put into your daily practice:

- Meditating, focusing on breathing
- Praying, focusing on gratitude and forgiveness
- Watching your Mind Movie, focusing on the exciting future that you are creating

You can even do the above list while you are at the gym! Close your eyes when you're on the spin bike and meditate. Watch your Mind Movie at the gym. Use what Tony Robbins calls and **NET** time. **No Extra Time.** I even write these books while I'm doing cardio at the gym. You have plenty of time to do this simple daily check-in.

## Weekly Schedule

Your weekly schedule is less motivational and more practical. Every week you want to focus on two main things:
1. your workout schedule
2. and your food prep.

Write out your plan. Make sure you understand where your workouts fit into your week. Know exactly what time and day you are performing each one. If you are meeting somebody for your exercise session, make sure you have confirmed the time with them in advance.

Prepping your food in advance is a great way to keep all your momentum and allow it to build. To do food prep, simply get a bunch of sealing containers. Think if your macronutrients. You want to cook a lot of protein, a lot of carbs, and make a huge salad. Divide each one of those up into smaller portions. At the end of your food prep you should have a bunch of little containers for each macronutrient.

At the start of each day, all you have to do is grab several containers and there you go.

Your weekly check-in is a great time to do all these things. I like doing my weekly work on Sunday because that seems to be the day that has the fewest obligations. However, if next Sunday looks busy, make a plan to do it on a different day.

## *Monthly Schedule*

Every month, choose an action that you want to turn into a habit. You can create so much lifetime momentum in just one month. Be sure to take 30 minutes or so to ask yourself the following questions:
- What positive habits have I created so far?
- How successful was I last month?
- What habits have I tried to create, yet haven't mastered yet?

- What is the one **_BIG habit_** that I will focus on in the coming month?

Quarterly schedule (every three months)

Every quarter, think about the types of workouts that you are doing and whether or not
1. you enjoy them, and
2. they are producing results as originally planned.

This is where you can do a complete overhaul of the type of workouts you're doing. Been doing Zumba for a while? Looking for a change? Maybe start lifting weights. Are your joints getting stiff from lifting too many weights? Maybe start doing Yoga or Pilates. Allow yourself the flexibility to completely change direction if needed.

When you start a specific workout style, make sure you give it at least three months before you assess progress. You will not necessarily see results in less time than that.

## *Yearly Schedule*

Every year, you want to brainstorm for at least a full day and brainstorm what your big picture goals are for your entire life. This is a great habit to get into and why I love January 1 so much. My process starts around Thanksgiving. At the end of November I start thinking about what next year will look like. I give myself a few weeks for my goals to ruminate in my head before I really start making these new habits.

I use a simple habits-based spreadsheet that I created in Google Sheets. Download it for free, add your big-picture yearly goals, then track your progress on a daily and weekly basis. Visit www.mycorebalance.com/go-to-the-gym to download that free resource.

# TIME TO GET STARTED

Now it's time for you to start developing your most important muscle, your consistency. Take it one day at a time, and then before you know it you will have years of positive fitness habits under your belt.

Right now you might feel overwhelmed. It's OK to feel like a complete beginner. The important thing is to just get started, even without knowing the full picture. Along the way, people will show up to help you just as you need them.

I'm here to help, too. Feel free to reach out with questions or comments. Text me at 408-883-4442.

I'm pushing you out of the nest now. It's time to fly. Go to the gym.

Your friend in health,

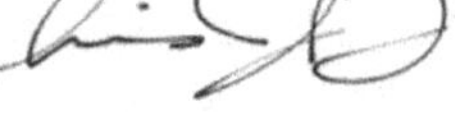

# OTHER BOOKS BY
# CHRIS JANKE-BUENO

## All available at Amazon.com

**Help! I Threw Out My Back**
Four Workouts to Ease Muscle Tension and
Develop Core Strength

**How to Build Muscle**
A Simple Approach to Getting Strong

**Help! My Diet Sucks!**
7 Simple Steps to Hone Your Healthy
Eating Habits Without the Diet Dogma,
Deprivation, and Dishonor - Whether You
Want To Lose, Gain, or Just Maintain